DIY Herbal Antibiotics And Antivirals

65 Natural Remedies Against Ailments Caused By Viruses, Bacteria And Other Disease-Causing Organisms

REGINA CRUZ

ISBN-13:978-1983990335

ISBN-10:1983990337

Disclaimer:

The information in this book is solely for informational purposes, not as a medical instruction to replace the advice of your physician or as a replacement for any treatment prescribed by your physician. The author and publisher do not take responsibility for any possible consequences from any treatment, procedure, exercise, dietary modification, action or application of medication which results from reading or following the information contained in this book.

If you are ill or suspect that you have a medical problem, we strongly encourage you to consult your medical, health, or other competent professional before adopting any of the suggestions in this book or drawing inferences from it.

This book and the author's opinions are solely for informational and educational purposes. The author specifically disclaims all responsibility for any liability, loss, or risk, personal or otherwise which is incurred as a consequence, directly or indirectly, of the use and application of any of the contents of this book

TABLE OF CONTENT

INTRODUCTION

An antibiotic and an antiviral are both medicines taken to
ward off illnesses and they do this by attacking the
infection. These infections, bacterial or viral, can either be
mild or severe. Viral infections and bacterial infections are
different but they are often mistaken for the other because
their symptoms are usually similar or in some cases, the
same.

There are a large number of antibiotics than antiviral. The
construction and make up of bacteria is relatively simpler
so drugs are easily developed to target them but antiviral
are not easily developed. As a matter of fact, they are
tricky, change frequently and mutate in semblance of its
original self. Resistance level of viruses is also quicker
than bacteria.

Additionally, ailments that are caused by viruses cannot be
cured quickly. They just hang in there until they run their
course or they are successfully fought off. In some cases,
the virus stays for a long time and wears the patient out.
Besides, a lingering virus may be due to some severe
conditions such as eczema, chronic fatigue and some form
of arthritis.

Why Herbal Remedy?

Herbal antiviral and antibiotic are natural means of helping an individual to ward off illness or disease. They both achieve this by targeting the cells that are generating the illness. They are more effective than traditional medicines in the following ways:

- Herbs are generally safe to use.

- Healing time is quicker.

- They are more effective in boosting the immune system.

- They do not present side effects especially when taken correctly.

- Their availability in mankind's natural environment for millions of years makes them dependable.

- Natural antiviral are much more powerful for treating viruses.

- Since most natural antiviral remedies have multiple uses, they also help in reliving the symptoms that come with the virus.

- Natural antibiotics are gentle on the system and extremely effective as well.

- These antibiotics do not merely contain the growth of the harmful bacteria but work to kill them off as well.

- Besides using them for treatment, they can also be used as prevention and this will totally eradicate the dependency on medical antibiotic and antiviral.

A Few Top Antibiotics And Antiviral Herbs

The following are some top natural herbs that fight viruses and bacteria in the human body. However, a lot of these herbs serve multiple functions as well.

<u>Blackberry</u> - is a blood purifier and the flu's no. 1 enemy. It works on bleeding gum when chewed. However, they shouldn't be taken regularly or on an empty stomach as they may lead to constipation and gastro intestinal disorders.

<u>Calendula or Marigold</u> - is effective against skin disease. It can be prepared in a number of ways including tincture, infusions, ointments and lotions.

<u>Chamomile</u> - It has anti inflammatory properties, treats nerve pain and rheumatism. It should not be infused for more than 5 minutes to avoid irritability and nausea.

<u>Cinnamon</u>- Has anti-bacterial properties and treat colds, alleviates abdominal pain as well as stomach cramps. To avoid vomiting and nausea, it should be used sparingly.

<u>Clove</u> - purifies the blood, since it induces sweating, it cures any type of cold as well. It also has anesthetic property and can be used to relieve toothache.

<u>Echinacea</u> - boosts the immune system, treats sore throat and common cold, fights typhoid fever, purifies the blood and speeds up the process of healing. It works excellently when taken as a tincture over an extensive period of time.

Garlic - is an excellent antibiotic with antiviral and antibacterial functions that effectively fights throat, nose and chest infections. It also kills intestinal parasites. Garlic is known for lowering blood sugar levels, blood pressure and cholesterol. However, it should be avoided by people with low blood pressure, stomach ulcer and gastritis.

It can be infused in oil, added to your diet or used as a tincture or capsule. Do not heat beyond 130 degrees if cooking because it will reduce its potency.

Linden - an old remedy against indigestion and sleeplessness, linden is effective against sore throat and cold but shouldn't be used regularly.

Mallow – as an excellent expectorant, mallow treats chest disorders of any kind. Boiling water should never be used on mallows because it tends to kill its healing properties. Instead, they should be covered with cold or lukewarm water and infused overnight.

Marjoram - a calming herb as well as a great liver tonic, it alleviates headache and also aids digestion. Additionally, it is a strong antioxidant with antiviral and antibacterial and helps to treat respiratory difficulties.

Marshmallow - has its antibacterial and antiviral properties as well as inflammatory effect that alleviate a range of irritation such as urinary disorders. To perverse its healing, it must also be infused in lukewarm or cold water.

Mint contains vitamin C, menthol and tannic acid. It works on the liver and eases nausea and vomiting. Furthermore, it alleviates flatulent colic and deals with insomnia and migraine.

Oregon Grape- this herb can be used to address viral infections to prevent them from developing into life-threatening bacterial infections. It has an anti-inflammatory property that is good for treating lung and respiratory infections. Skin conditions such as eczema, acne and psoriasis are also dealt with. It also helps in maintaining a healthy liver function.

Nettle an excellent blood purifier, it also fights anemia and ensures a good circulation. It is also effective against rheumatism, asthma, arthritis and scurvy. It can be used as a conditioner for very greasy hair.

Thyme has antiseptic, antispasmodic, antimicrobial and antioxidant, properties. It kills intestinal parasites and treats respiratory problems.

Astragalus - effective for boosting the immune system, it is also used for treating more serious conditions such as heart diseases.

Mullein - Mullein is an effective expectorant and an antispasmodic agent that can dissolve phlegm. It provides relief from earache when its flowers are infused in olive oil for 3 weeks.

Sage has powerful antibacterial, antiviral and antiseptic properties. It alleviates sore throat and deals with any kind of pain related to menstruation. However, sage shouldn't be taken regularly because they can lead to muscle constriction.

Elder (elderberries and elderflowers), a gentle laxative, also improve the immune system, reduce coughing and asthma. However, elderberries should never be eaten fresh.

Prickly ash bark is one very powerful antiviral. It is good for depression, chronic infections, and digestive ailments that come with long-term viruses. 1 to3 drops of tincture thrice a day is the ideal treatment. It shouldn't be used by breastfeeding mothers.

Ginger- a great antiviral remedy, ginger helps to treat various kinds of infections like cough, cold and strep throat, cold. The ginger herb is easy to use and can be adopted for a range of remedies.

Apple Cider Vinegar - offer various benefits such as soothing stomach upsets and sore throats, fighting diabetes, itches as well as brightening the skin and providing healthier hair.

Oil Of Oregano – a serious antiviral, oil oregano can be taken internally on externally on affected skin.

Licorice is antibacterial and antiviral. It is generally used for gastric ulcers.

Honey- a delicious sweetener that soothes the throat contains 3 powerful vitamins: A, C, and E. it has antiseptic, antibacterial, and antiviral properties.

<u>Lemon and Orange</u> -Citrus fruits all have antibacterial, antiviral and antiseptic properties so they are helpful against cold and infections.

<u>Lemon Balm</u>- Lemon balm has antiviral properties and is a powerful antihistamine. It prevents tumors development and lowers blood pressure.

<u>St. John's Wort</u>- this is a great immune system booster and virus fighter.

Safety& Preparatory Tips
<u>Safety</u>

- Herbs may treat minor disorders but if you suspect some complications, immediately consult your doctor. Let your doctor know about any herbal remedies you may be taking especially if you are under medication to avoid problems that may arise from double medication.
- On no account should you stop taking a prescribed medicine without professional consultation.
- Pregnant and breastfeeding mothers must seek their doctor's consent before using any herb.
- Do not pick herbs in the wild if you cannot positively identify them, so you don't mistakenly gather poisonous plants.
- Suspicious herbs should simply be discarded. This is because some herbs are hallucinogenic,

addictive, carcinogenic or abortive. Some are for external applications only.

- Store completely dried and crushed plants in an airtight glass containers and keep away from direct sunlight and heat.
- Products must be labeled correctly. Specify the preparation name, its purpose, processing date, the amount to take, the ingredients and any adverse effects on the container.
- Check out the freshness, quality and origin of dried herbs before buying. This will help you to avoid products that are not grown organically as they are usually without packaging date or usage by date.
- Transfer the bought herb immediately to a jar and label it specifying the name and purchase date.
- Regularly check your products and throw them away at any sign of mould. Use them for composting after a year.
- Do not delay. Use natural treatments immediately the problem occurs so the infection doesn't worsen. They can also be taken as a preventative remedy.
- Listen to your body to be sure of correct herb, dosage and frequency that suits you. Certain herbs or even recipes may cause disagreements. For instance, digested garlic may cause stomach cramps or heartburn for certain individuals. Additionally, fennel seeds make one sweat. Certain individuals may be uncomfortable with the strong smell that comes with this sweat.

- Ideally, treatment shouldn't last more than 3 weeks.

<u>Preparatory</u>

- Hygiene is imperative. Boil equipments such as jars and bottles for about 15 minutes before you begin.
- Herbal teas are easy to make. It only requires a cup, hot water and a method to steep your tea. Simply steep a tbsp of the preferred herb in a teapot of very hot water for 3-10 minutes. For children, use 1 tsp herbs in the same amount of water.
- Cover it so it doesn't evaporate too quickly. It is better to use a glass or porcelain teapot when making teas. Be sure to rinse the teapot with hot water. Do not take more than 4 cups of tea daily unless contraindicated.
- When making decoctions, use a lidded glass or enameled pan.
- The quantity of herb is important during infusion. For dried herbs, use 1 teaspoon per cup of hot water but double this amount for fresh herbs.
- For capsules and syrups take one or two capsules or tablespoon every 3to 4 hours for the initial 3 days then reduce the amount.
- Cover tinctures with alcohol to ensure complete extract of natural properties and to preserve its freshness.

- Lastly, do not forget that herbal tea can be refrigerated for 3 days; that cordials last longer than syrups and that herbs in capsule remain fresh in small dark containers for at least 3 months.

HERBAL TEAS

Turmeric Tea

Turmeric has antibiotic, antiviral, antioxidant and anti-inflammatory benefits.

Ingredients

4 mugs water

1 teaspoon turmeric, ground

1 teaspoon ginger (optional)

Lemon and/ or honey, to taste

Preparation

1. Bring water to a boil. Add the turmeric and let it simmer gently for about 10 minutes.

2. Using a fine sieve, strain the tea into a mug. Season the tea with lemon and/or honey.

3. If using, add a teaspoon of ginger.

Sage Tea

Strong medicinal tea

Ingredients

2 heaped tbsp fresh or dried sage

4cups water

Preparation

1. Place sage in a saucepan of water. Bring to a boil and then simmer for at least 15 minutes.

2. Remove from heat. Let it cool for 15 minutes. Strain it and store in the refrigerator.

3. Reheat to drink or take cold, if preferred. If desired, add a little maple syrup or honey to taste.

Pectoral Flowers Tea

Bronchitis and cough if not properly treated may become chronic. Pectoral Flowers are extremely effective and have been proven by research to have no side effects.

Ingredients

1 tsp mullein

1 tsp corn poppy

1 tsp marshmallow

1 tsp plantain

1 tsp linden

1 tsp violet

½ tsp thyme

Preparation

1. Place marshmallow aside. Pour 4 cups boiling water over the rest of the flowers.

2. Leave to infuse for about 3 minutes then strain.

3. When tea is cold or lukewarm, add the marshmallow, leaving to stand overnight.

4. Strain again and heat the tea once more.

5. Add the lemon juice, sweeten with honey and drink.

6. If cough is severe, take a cup of tea every 3-4 hours.

Magic Tea

Contains powerful ingredients to soothe your mind and body

Ingredients

1 tbsp sweet violet

1 tbsp marjoram

1 tbsp basil

1 tbsp rose petals

1 tbsp crushed rosehips

½ Vanilla pod, cut lengthwise

1 tsp orange peel

½ tsp of grated Ginger

½ tsp aniseeds

2 tbsp fresh or dried berries

Preparation

1. Begin by softening the dry berries in a little water then put 4 cups water to boil.

2. Place the rosehips in a pan and immediately add the boiling water. Leave it to boil for about 10 minutes.

3. Turn off heat. Add the marjoram, rose petals, aniseeds, violet, orange peel and ginger.

4. Infuse the herbs for 3-5 minutes then strain the tea.

5. Scrap the inside of the cut vanilla pod in the teapot.

6. Strain the berries and then add the stained liquid to the tea.

7. Put few berries in each cup then pour the tea.

8. Drink hot in winter and icy cold in summer. It works on your body and mind like magic!

Tomato Tea

For all sinus issues

Ingredients

2 cups tomato juice

2 tbsp lemon juice

3 garlic, crushed

Hot sauce (cayenne pepper, black pepper, dried pepper flakes or fresh hot pepper)

Preparation

1. Combine ingredients and heat on low for 10 minutes.

2. sip slowly, allowing the tea to sit in the back of throat.

3. Suck the hot fumes through the sinuses and down into the lungs.

4. Drink as needed until all trace of infection disappears.

Digestive Tea For The Liver
Alleviate discomfort, ensures good digestion

Ingredients

½ tsp fennel seeds

½ tsp caraway seeds

1 tbsp crushed rosehips

1 tbsp mint

1 tbsp linden

1 tbsp elderberry syrup in each cup

(See recipe below)

Preparation

1. Crush seeds slightly. Boil 4 cups of water for 3 minutes. Infuse the seeds and the herbs into the boiling water.

 2. Add 1 tbsp of elderberry in each cup and pour the tea over it.

3. Take 1 cup at least 1 hour before or after meal.

Recipe For Elderberry Syrup

Ingredients

5 cups elderberry, crushed

1 Lemon juice

Honey or raw Sugar

<u>Preparation</u>

1. Place elderberries in a pan, cover with water and boil.

2. Add the lemon juice and leave to stand for 24 hours. Strain and measure then bring to boil.

3. Warm the same amount of raw sugar or honey in a saucepan.

4. Add the tea and boil again, simmering and stirring regularly until it becomes syrupy.

Bad Breath Tea

<u>Ingredients</u>

1 tsp myrrh powder

¼ tsp goldenseal powder

2 sprigs parsley, coarsely chopped

3 cloves

2 cups water

<u>Preparation</u>

1. Bring water to boil in a pan.

2. Add cloves, goldenseal, parsley and myrrh to it. Steep for up to10 minutes and leave to cool.

3. Use this tea to rinse your mouth.

Cleansing Tea

For bright eyes, clear skin and shiny hair

<u>Ingredients</u>

1 tbsp calendula flowers

1 tbsp nettle

1 tbsp linden

1 tbsp peppermint

½ tbsp dandelion flowers and chamomile flowers

<u>Preparation</u>

1. Bring 4 cups of water to boil. Immediately infuse the herbs and flowers in it for 3-5 minutes.

2. If using externally, leave to cool for 15 minutes.

3. Strain tea and utilize as needed.

Anti- Bloating Tea

<u>Ingredients</u>

1 tsp fennel seed, crushed

1 cup water

<u>Preparation</u>

1. Combine ingredients in a pot. Cover and bring to boil on low heat.

2. Let it steep for 10 minutes. Leave to cool and then strain.

3. Take 2 cups daily.

Winter Delight Tea

To prevent cold and flu

<u>Ingredients</u>

1 tbsp cooked elderberries and elderflowers,

1 tbsp Echinacea leaves and roots

1 tbsp raspberry leaves

½ cup dried Apples pieces

½ tsp cinnamon

1 tsp orange peel

1 tbsp rosehip syrup in each cup

(See recipe below)

<u>Preparation</u>

1. Begin by softening the fruit in a little water. Boil elder berries.

2. Pour 1litre of boiling over the boiled elder berries, elderflowers, raspberry leaves and Echinacea.

3. Leave for 10 minutes add the orange peel and the cinnamon. Let it stand five minutes then strain.

4. Next, strain the fruit and add the liquid to tea and heat tea again.

5. In each cup, put pieces of apple and 1 tablespoon of rosehip syrup.

6. Pour tea and drink hot. Enjoy it as desired.

<u>Recipe For Rosehip Syrup</u>

<u>Ingredients</u>

5 cups rosehip, crushed

1 lemon juice

Honey or raw Sugar

<u>Preparation</u>

1. Place rosehip in a pan, cover with water and boil.

2. Add the lemon juice and leave to stand for 24 hours. Strain and measure then bring to boil.

3. Warm the same amount of raw sugar or honey in a saucepan.

4. Add the tea and boil again, simmering and stirring regularly until it becomes really syrupy

Lemon Balm Sun Tea

<u>Ingredients</u>

2 tbsp fresh leaves or 1 heaping tbsp dried leaves

Lemon juice/ honey

1cup water

<u>Preparation</u>

1. Place the lemon balm and cool water in a jar. Cover and leave in the sun for 3-4 hours.

2. Strain liquid, add lemon juice and/or honey

3. Add mint for a lemony minty tea.

Tea To Fight Chickenpox

<u>Ingredients</u>

1 tbsp holy basil or chamomile herb

Lemon

Cinnamon

Honey

<u>Preparation</u>

1. Put herb in boiling water. Allow it to steep for 5-10 minutes and then strain.

2. Add a little lemon, honey or cinnamon. Gently sip

3. Drink tea several times daily.

Anti- Asthma Tea

…To ease asthma attack. Oregano contains compounds that help in cleansing the respiratory tract and bronchial tubes.

<u>Preparation</u>

1. 1. Bring water to boil

2. Place oregano herb in the boiling water and cover for 10 minutes.

3. Strain off and add honey.

4. Drink tea hot four to five times daily.

Another option - extract juice from oregano leaves then take1 tablespoon hourly to relieve chronic coughs and asthma.

Anti-Allergic Tea

For treatment of hay-fever and hives

<u>Ingredients</u>

1tbsp nettles

2 tsp sage leaf

1tbsp elder flower

¼ tsp peppermint

2 tsp eyebright

Honey (optional)

<u>Preparation</u>

1. Bring 1 large cup of water to boil.

2. Place all ingredients in the boiled water and cover for 10 minutes.

3. Strain off and add honey if using.

4. Sip tea while still hot, taking one dose daily for at least 3days

Cold Flu Tea

<u>Ingredients</u>

3 cups water

1/2 teaspoon elder flowers

1/2 teaspoon yarrow flowers

1/2 teaspoon Peppermint leaves

1/2 teaspoon Schisandra berries

1/2 teaspoon Echinacea root

<u>Preparation</u>

1. Bring the water to a boil. Place all the herbs in a teapot then immediately pour the boiling water over them.

2. Steep for a 20- 30 minutes. Next, strain it and drink all through the day.

3. You could make two batches and keep one batch in the refrigerator but warm before drinking.

SOLUTIONS

Garlic-Honey Vinegar
Cures throat and lung infections. Soothes coughing as well

<u>Ingredients</u>

5-10 cloves of garlic, raw& chopped

Apple cider vinegar

Raw honey, to taste

<u>Preparation</u>

1. Get a jar. Put the apple cider vinegar in it and add the garlic.

2. Leave it to soak overnight.

3. Add raw honey and take spoonfuls all through the day.

Gout Herbal Treatment
Apple Cider Vinegar is acidic and this helps to relieve acute pain in gout while honey increases the body's anti-inflammatory response.

<u>Ingredients</u>

1tsp apple cider vinegar

2 tbsp honey

<u>Preparation</u>

Mix and take twice daily, in the morning and at night shortly before bedtime.

Turmeric & Milk Solution

Treats internal and external problems of the body

<u>Ingredients</u>

½ tsp of turmeric powder

1 cup hot milk

2 tsp honey

Pinch black pepper

<u>Preparation</u>

1. Add turmeric powder onto the cup of hot milk.

2. Add honey and black pepper to it.

3. Stir thoroughly, add milk and drink hot.

Garlic Lemonade

Drink daily throughout the duration of illness

<u>Ingredients</u>

2-3 lemons

3-4 fresh ginger, sliced

2-4 garlic cloves, chopped

Raw honey

Water

<u>Preparation</u>

1. Combine garlic and fresh ginger in a 1 quart mason container.

2. Cover it and let it steep for 20- 30 minutes.

3. Add juice of lemons and honey to taste (about ¼ cup).

4. Leave herbs in mixture or strain.

5. Take warm and as needed.

Ginger Root For Gout

<u>Ingredients</u>

1part fenugreek powder

1 part dried ginger root powder

1 part turmeric powder

<u>Preparation</u>

1. Combine all ingredients and add warm water to it.

2. Mix thoroughly. Take 1tsp two times daily

Ginger Remedy

For Indigestion

<u>Ingredients</u>

2 tsp ginger juice

1 tsp lemon juice

Pinch of salt

Pinch of black salt

<u>Preparation</u>

1. Combine all ingredients thoroughly.

2. Take with or without water.

Anti- Gas Asafetida Remedy

<u>Ingredients</u>

Pinch of asafetida

Pinch salt

½ tsp ginger powder

1 cup lukewarm water

<u>Preparation</u>

Combine all ingredients. Drink everyday for relief from gas problem.

BALMS AND OINTMENTS

Multi-Purpose Healing Balm
Works on bruises, diaper rash, burns, bruises and muscle pain.

<u>Ingredients</u>

8 oz Shea butter

2 tbsp comfrey

2 tbsp calendula petals, tightly packed

6 oz coconut oil (after immersing herbs, add adequate coconut oil back in so it equals 14 oz once more).

1 tbsp marshmallow root, tightly packed

1 tbsp yarrow

1 tbsp arnica, tightly packed

1 tbsp plantain

2 tbsp beeswax

20 drops lemon essential oil

20 drops wild orange essential oil

10 drops frankincense essential oil

5 drops lavender essential oil

5 drops melaleuca essential oil

1 tbsp vitamin e acetate oil

<u>Preparation</u>

1. Preheat oven to 200 degrees. Melt Shea butter and coconut oil in a pan on the stovetop

2. Next, add the herbs, stirring them in then transfer pan to oven. Allow it to steep there for 4- 5 hours.

3. Strain the infused oil into a container. Add the coconut oil until the weight of all the oils is equal to 14 ounce once more.

4. Rinse pan and pour the oils back into the pan. Warm the infused pan, add beeswax and stir until it is melted.

5. Take out from heat, add the vitamin E oil and essential oils and stir.

6. Pour into a lidded clean container or a pint size jar, label and store in a cool, dark place.

7. Apply it few times daily.

No- Diaper Rash Oil Treatment

<u>Ingredients</u>

¼ cup witch hazel solution

1½ tsp organic grape-seed oil

½ tsp lavender oil

½ tsp tea tree oil

½ tsp chamomile oil

½ tsp geranium oil

<u>Preparation</u>

1. Combine all ingredients in a glass bottle.

2. Store in a cool place

3. Use sparingly when changing baby's diaper

Cayenne Skin Remedy

For skin disorders such as eczema and psoriasis

<u>Ingredients</u>

¾ cup cayenne pepper, chopped

21/4 cups olive oil

<u>Preparation</u>

1. In the top of a double boiler, place cayenne pepper in olive oil. Add water to the bottom of the double boiler until it is full. Place over low heat.

2. Let the cayenne mixture simmer for about 3 hours then take it out from heat.

3. Leave to cool at room temperature.

3. Pass through a fine-mesh strainer. Transfer into a dark, glass jar.

4. Massage into the skin at least three times daily.

Arnica Salve

As an anti-inflammatory herb, Arnica is effective and helps in reducing swelling from black eye as well as treat bruises, sprains and muscle soreness.

<u>Ingredients</u>

1 ounce dried arnica herb

1 cup olive oil

1.5 ounce beeswax

2-3 wintergreen essential oil

1 jar with cover

Small storage container (tin or jam jar)

<u>Preparation</u>

1. Place dried herb in a jar

2. Pour olive oil over it then cover and store for 6 weeks but be sure to shake the jar daily.

3. In a double boiler, warm the oil. Add the beeswax stirring until it melts. Next, add the essential oil.

4. Pour the salve into a tin or jam jar

5. Leave to cool. Apply the salve to the affected area 2 to 3 times daily.

Honey & Clove for Scabies

Clove oil can be very irritating to skin, so do a test patch before applying to a wide area.

<u>Ingredients</u>

10 drops of clove oil

1 cup vegetable oil or

1/2 cup of honey &1/2 cup water mixture

<u>Preparation</u>

1. Apply a generous portion to the affected area and leave overnight.

Oregano Chest Rub
For Whooping Cough

<u>Ingredients</u>

15 drops oregano oil

1 ounce jojoba, almond or olive oil

<u>Preparation</u>

1. Combine ingredients and shake thoroughly to mix

2. Rub on chest before bedtime

REMEDIES FROM EVERYDAY INGREDIENTS

Eggshell Wonder
For ingrown toenails and blisters

<u>Preparation</u>

1. Crack 1 egg and tear off pieces of the egg membrane

2. Wet them and place on affected area.

3. Use a bandage if necessary.

Potato Remedy
For swollen dark eyes

Potato contains enzymes that assist in dispersing the old blood that comes from a bruise.

<u>Preparation</u>

1. Cut 1 potato into thin slices

2. Put these slices in the refrigerator so it becomes cold.

3. Once cold, remove from refrigerator, place these cold slices on your eye and the surrounding skin for about 15 minutes.

4. Alternatively, grate 1 potato and place on the eye or apply potato juice using a cotton ball around your eye.

Plantain Application
For Earache

<u>Ingredients</u>

10 fresh plantain leaves, crushed

1 cup olive oil

<u>Preparation</u>

1. Put the crushed plantain leaves in a jar. Pour olive oil over them.

2. Close the jar very tightly so no air penetrates. Store in a dark place for 3weeks, shaking regularly.

3. Gently strain the oil then pour into small sterilized bottles.

4. Drop a few drops in a cotton ball and place on the ear.

5. Use as often as needed but see a doctor if pain persists.

Tomato Facial Mask

For stubborn acne

<u>Ingredients</u>

1 tomato

<u>Preparation</u>

1. Cut an 'x' at the tomato top with a knife then run it under warm water for 2 minutes.

2. Peel off the already soft skin (on account of the warm water used). Deseed the tomato and mash up the pulp.

3. Turn pulp into a paste, mix thoroughly and then apply as facial mask for 1 hour

4. Rinse face thoroughly.

Carrot/ Potato Remedy

For reddened skin

<u>Ingredients</u>

1 carrot, boiled and mashed

1 potato, boiled and mashed

1 tbsp, ground oatmeal

<u>Preparation</u>

1. Combine ingredients. Let it cool to room temperature

2. Apply all over the face and leave for 30 minutes

3. Wash off with warm water.

Plantain Poultice

Ingredients

Fresh plantain leaves, mashed

Preparation

Wet the mashed plantain leaves and apply on stings or insect bites for fast relief when outdoors.

Guava Leaves Compress

For recurrent sty Infection

Preparation

1. Wash a few guava leaves and make a compress

2. Apply on affected area

Salt Water Compress

Extremely helpful remedy for conjunctivitis

<u>Preparation</u>

1. Add 1 tablespoon salt to boiling water. Mix well and dip a cotton ball in it.

2. Apply on affected area.

CAPSULES AND TINCTURES

Eggshell Capsules

Perfect antacids for stomach cramp relief. Good source of calcium too!

Ingredients

12 egg shells

Empty capsules

Preparation

1. Place shells on the oven tray. Bake until they are brown.

2. Leave them to cool completely then grind them finely in a coffee grinder.

3. Fill capsules up. Take two capsules thrice daily for three days.

4. Use occasionally so it doesn't cause constipation

Antibiotic Capsule Remedy

Ingredients

1 tbsp Thyme &Elder berries

1 tsp Cloves

1 tsp Garlic powder

1 tbsp Echinacea tincture

Empty capsules

<u>Preparation</u>

1. Put the spices and herbs in your coffee grinder.

2. Grind until they form fine powder.

3. Fill the capsules up. At the first symptoms, take 2 capsules every three hours for three days. Afterwards, take two capsules thrice daily all through the rest of the week.

Fast Relief Antibiotic Tincture
<u>Ingredients</u>

1 tbsp Echinacea roots, Thyme, Mallow,

Mullein Elderberry and Plantain,

3 crushed cloves

3 cloves garlic, sliced

1 tbsp ginger, grated

Fruit alcohol, Gin or Vodka

<u>Preparation</u>

1. Put herbs and spices in a lidded glass jar and cover with alcohol.

2. Leave jar on the windowsill for 3 weeks. Shake it often.

3. Strain and fill small sterilized bottles up.

4. Dilute 30 drops of it in a hot drink with honey and lemon juice.

5. Take it four times daily for three days and afterwards three times daily for a week.

Toothache Cure With Prickly Ash

<u>Ingredients</u>

Prickly ash

Vodka or alcohol

<u>Preparation</u>

1. Take a small amount of Prickly Ash tincture and immerse in a cotton wad until it is soaked.

2. Hold it directly against the sore tooth. Result is usually experience within minutes.

3. Alternatively, take some Prickly Ash herb powder and sprinkle it on a small piece of peanut-butter coated white bread (the peanut butter is to help hold to it in place). Mould bread around the tooth.

Remedy For Saliva Loss

For very dry mouth and non-functional salivary glands

<u>Preparation</u>

1. Take some prickly ash tincture or powder. Place onto the tongue and let it stay in the mouth until it is absorbed.

2. Do this every few hours. A significant improvement will be obtained.

Glue Ear Treatment

<u>Ingredients</u>

3-6 drops Echinacea

Alcohol

<u>Preparation</u>

1. Make an Echinacea tincture. Add ½ teaspoon of water to it.

2. Dry into the affected ear 2 times daily.

3. The alcohol content that is in the tinctures enables the mucus to dry out while the Echinacea kills off the bad bugs.

Acute Cold & Chronic Infection Treatment

Echinacea tincture or

Echinacea Capsule

<u>Preparation</u>

1. Take 1 tsp of tincture every 1-3 hours or 1-2 capsules every 2-3 hours for the first two days.

2. Reduce dosage to 2 tsp tincture or 6 capsules daily.

3. For a chronic infection, take 1/2 tsp tincture or 2 capsules thrice daily for three weeks.

4. Abstain for a week before continuing.

Winter Echinacea Tincture

<u>Ingredients</u>

3/4 fresh Echinacea herb or1/2 dried herb

80 or 100 proof vodka

<u>Preparation</u>

1. Fill herb to the top with vodka

2. Leave to sit for 3-6 weeks, shaking daily

3. Strain and squeeze out every drop. Compost the left over herb material.

4. To make an herbal extract that contains no alcohol, use food-grade vegetable glycerin and mix 50% with distilled water.

HERBAL MOUTHWASH

The Aloe Vera Intervention
For mouth ulcers

<u>Ingredient</u>

Aloe Vera Juice

<u>Preparation</u>

1. Rinse the mouth with aloe Vera juice 3-4 times daily.

2. Canker sores are most excruciating in the first 3 to 4 days but disappear in about 10 days.

Sage Gargle
For sore throat

<u>Ingredients</u>

2 teaspoons dried or fresh Sage leaves

1 cup boiling water

1/4 ounce salt

<u>Preparation</u>

1. Pour boiling water over the sage. Cover it and let it steep for 20 minutes.

2. Strain, add salt and gargle as needed.

3. It can be refrigerated for a few days.

Halitosis Gargle

<u>Ingredients</u>

½ tbsp cinnamon

½ tsp-1 tsp baking soda

2 lemons, squeezed

11/2 tsp honey

1 cup warm water

<u>Preparation</u>

1. Put the cinnamon into a tight fitting lidded jar.

2. Add juice of lemon and honey to it. Add baking soda and honey.

3. Pour warm water into the jar to melt the honey. Stir thoroughly.

4. Shake before use, gargle for 1 minute with 2 tbsp.

Lemon Throat Spray

Ingredients

15 drops Lemon essential oil

1/4 cup water

1/4 cup lemon juice

5 drops Peppermint essential oil

Preparation

1. Combine ingredients and pour mixture into a spray bottle.

2. Shake thoroughly then spray gently into the throat all through the day.

Saline Gargle

Helps to remove mucus from respiratory tube caused by bacteria or viral infection

Ingredients

1-2 tbsp salt

1 glass water

Pinch turmeric powder

Preparation

1. Bring water to boil. Stir thoroughly and add the turmeric powder.

2. Leave for few minutes to cool.

3. Take 1 swig of the warm water and gargle for 1 to 2 minutes

4. Swig and gargle four to five times daily

Quick Relief For Canker Sores

For those who can stand the bitter taste of this herb, the relief is almost instantaneous.

<u>Ingredients</u>

A fresh piece of Sorrel herb

<u>Preparation</u>

1. Take the piece of this herb, hold against the canker sores, and keep holding until they become soggy.

2. Remove after about 1 minute and repeat the process.

HERBAL SYRUPS &TONICS

Sugar Onion Cough Syrup
Ingredients

2–3 onions, peeled and chopped

Brown or white sugar

Preparation

1. Get a sterilized glass jar. Alternate half inch layers of sugar and then onion in it. Start with the sugar and end with it as well.

2. Keep it refrigerated overnight.

3. Leave onions in the syrup or strain out._Keep refrigerated.

Garlic Honey
Ingredients

1/4 cup raw honey

6 cloves raw garlic, finely grated

Preparation

1. Let the grated raw honey sit for a bout10 minutes to trigger medicinal compounds.

2. Add the honey to garlic, stir thoroughly to mix. Store it in a sealed and dry jar.

3. Before taking, use a dry and clean spoon to stir and turn the jar to mix well.

Take content immediately.

Cough &Sore Throat Syrup
<u>Ingredients</u>

1/2 cup licorice root

1 cup fennel seed

1/2 cup valerian root

1/2 cup slippery elm bark

1/4 cup cinnamon bark

1/2 cup wild cherry bark

1/8 cup ginger root

1 and 1/2 tsp orange peel, dried

1 cup raw honey or maple syrup

2 drops peppermint or spearmint essential oil

<u>Preparation</u>

1. Combine about one cup of herb mixture (two ounces) with 1 quart of water.

2. Place on low heat to simmer until 1 pint of liquid is left.

3. Strain herbs from liquid. Pour back the liquid into the pot.

4. Add maple syrup or honey and then warm the sweetened mixture so it mixes well.

5. Add the essential oil.

6. Take out from heat, pour into bottle and label.

7. If refrigerated, this will last for many weeks or even months.

8. Usage: take 1-2 tsp every hour daily or whenever you feel a cough coming on.

Yellow Onion &Honey Syrup

<u>Ingredients</u>

1 yellow onion, medium size, thinly slice

1-2 cups raw, unfiltered honey

<u>Preparation</u>

1. Lay the sliced onion in the glass jar. Pour honey over it and loosely place all the onion into the jar.

2. Fill jar with honey to the onion level. Leave overnight or for 8 hours.

3. Carefully strain the onion pieces. This remedy makes about 1 cup.

Blackberry Tonic

<u>Ingredients</u>

Fights flu and tastes just great!

9 pounds blackberries

2 quarts water

1 lemon juice

6 ½ cup raw sugar

<u>Preparation</u>

1. Crush the berries. Cover with water and leave them to stand for 24 hours.

2. Boil the mixture. Using muslin, wring out the pulp to strain.

3. Put sugar into the saucepan along with the juice and allow it to boil for 15 minutes.

4. Simmer until it thickens.

5. Fill sterilized bottles up

MISCELLANEOUS

Flaxseed Therapy

Effective for eye infections but should never be used by pregnant women.

<u>Ingredients</u>

1 ounce flaxseed, bruised

½ cup water

<u>Preparation</u>

1. Put half cup of water to boil. Once boiled, add the bruised flax seed.

2. Leave the mixture in the hot water for 15- 20 minutes.

3. Pass the mixture through a strainer to strain excess water.

4. Get a clean washcloth; place the warm flaxseed onto it. Apply directly to the eye.

5. Repeat three times on a daily basis until the symptoms disappear.

Horseradish Poultice Therapy

Although arthritis can be incapacitating, herbal remedies can considerably reduce pain sensations so that life becomes more enjoyable for individuals who have painful joints.

Fresh horseradish root

<u>Preparation</u>

1. Add lots of water and the horseradish root in a blender, process until it makes a thick paste.

2. Soak a piece of cotton fabric in hot water. Spread the processed horseradish root mixture onto the cloth. Cover it with another layer of dry cotton fabric.

3. Next, place the moist area of the poultice over the sore joint. Leave on for about 30 minutes. Keep it hot by placing a hot water bottle on the poultice. Remove poultice if it gets uncomfortable.

4. Since the heat will increase circulation in the area affected, the skin will redden. This is normal.

Herbal Hair Care

Indian lilac or neem has antibacterial and antiseptic properties for dandruff, scalp acne, itchy scalp, hair fall.

<u>Preparation</u>

1. Boil some neem leaves. Leave to cool

2. Pass the solution through a strainer.

3. Use as hair rinse two or three times in a week.

Homemade Hand Sanitizer

<u>Ingredients</u>

1tbsp witch hazel extract

10 drops lavender essential oil

10 drops tea tree essential oil

8 drops lemongrass essential oil

8 drops rosemary essential oil

5 drops eucalyptus essential oil

¼ aloe Vera gel or lotion

<u>Preparation</u>

Combine all ingredients. Transfer to a pumped glass jar.

Another Hand Sanitizer

<u>Ingredients</u>

1 tsp. aloe Vera gel

3 oz. filtered water

10 drops cinnamon essential oil

20 drops lemon essential oil

10 drops rosemary essential oil

10 drops clove essential oil

10 drops eucalyptus essential oil

<u>Preparation</u>

1. Combine ingredients in a spray dispenser. Shake gently and spray 3-5 times onto the hands.

2. Massage into hands for 10 seconds.

Herbal Steam

Blocked nasal and bronchial passages respond to warm, moist open air. The entire house can also be humidified and disinfected by simmering the water with essential oils or herbs on low heat for 30 minutes.

<u>Ingredients</u>

3 cups water

5 drops Lavender essential oil

5 drops Rosemary essential oil

5 drops Bergamot essential oil

<u>Preparation</u>

1. Pour water to pan and bring to a simmer. Take it out from heat and add the essential oils.

2. Cover head with a bath towel and hold your face over the steam. Tuck the towel ends around the pan to prevent the steam from escaping.

3. Breathe in the scented steam as deeply as possible, emerging for fresh air every 1-2 minutes.

Garlic Feet

For bad cough and chest colds

<u>Ingredients</u>

Garlic cloves, crushed

Olive oil

<u>Preparation</u>

1. Crush the garlic cloves and place inside a small jar or bowl. Cover in olive oil for 30 minutes.

2. Rub on feet. The garlic pieces may also be placed between the toes.

3. Put socks on and leave overnight.

4. Do not be surprised if you have garlic breath in the morning. This indicates its effectiveness. Garlic goes inside the system and heads directly for the lungs.

Essential Oil Vapor Rub

- Antibiotic and antiviral

- stimulates blood circulation thereby reducing constriction

-relieve congestion and kill infection

<u>Ingredients</u>

3 drops Thyme essential oil

10 drops Eucalyptus essential oil

1/8 cup Olive oil

10 drops Peppermint essential oil

<u>Preparation</u>

1. Combine all ingredients. Rub on chest and throat.

2. Rub oil briskly onto the skin in order to increase the warmth of the balm

3. Place a warm piece of cloth or flannel on the chest to immediately increase the warming sensation.

Warts Eliminator

<u>Ingredients</u>

2 tbsp apple cider vinegar

Piece of cotton cloth or cotton balls

Bandage or gauze

<u>Preparation</u>

1. Soak cotton cloth or balls in apple cider vinegar.

2. Let it saturate for a while then press out excess liquid gently.

3. Place over wart and secure with a bandage, cloth or gauze.

4. Do this every night for 1 to 2 weeks. Warts should die and then come off.

Marigold Anti- Itch Paste

To reduce chickenpox itch

2tbsp marigold flowers

1tsp hazel leaves

1 cup water

<u>Preparation</u>

1. Mix herbs together. Place the mixture in water and leave to sit overnight.

2. Grind mixture well the next morning

3. Rub paste directly on rashes.

4. Leave it there for at least 1 hour.

5. Wash off with water then pat dry gently.